El Amine Cheroual

Bisphenol A

AF571172

El Amine Cheroual

Bisphenol A

Environmental and food contamination, health risks and alternative solutions

ScienciaScripts

Imprint

Any brand names and product names mentioned in this book are subject to trademark, brand or patent protection and are trademarks or registered trademarks of their respective holders. The use of brand names, product names, common names, trade names, product descriptions etc. even without a particular marking in this work is in no way to be construed to mean that such names may be regarded as unrestricted in respect of trademark and brand protection legislation and could thus be used by anyone.

Cover image: www.ingimage.com

This book is a translation from the original published under ISBN 978-613-9-54523-0.

Publisher:
Sciencia Scripts
is a trademark of
Dodo Books Indian Ocean Ltd. and OmniScriptum S.R.L publishing group

120 High Road, East Finchley, London, N2 9ED, United Kingdom
Str. Armeneasca 28/1, office 1, Chisinau MD-2012, Republic of Moldova, Europe
Managing Directors: Ieva Konstantinova, Victoria Ursu
info@omniscriptum.com

Printed at: see last page
ISBN: 978-620-8-51286-6

Copyright © El Amine Cheroual
Copyright © 2024 Dodo Books Indian Ocean Ltd. and OmniScriptum S.R.L publishing group

FOREWORD

Since the invention of metal cans by Nicolas Appert in 1810, their use has spread throughout the world, transforming food preservation. Every year, almost 302 billion cans are produced and sold worldwide. Their popularity is due to the many advantages they offer the food industry: effective protection against external spoilage agents, long shelf life, and ease of transport and storage at ambient temperature.

However, the risk of corrosion inside these cans, particularly in the presence acidic foods such as fruit and vegetables, has led manufacturers to coat them with an epoxy-phenol resin lining. This coating is designed to prevent direct contact between the food and the metal, thereby reducing the risk of contamination by substances derived from the metal. This resin is mainly obtained by polymerising bisphenol A (BPA), a toxic chemical compound also used in other materials in contact with food, such as polycarbonate plastics, paper and polyvinyl chloride.

BPA, a synthetic substance in the family of aromatic organic compounds, consists of two hydroxyphenol groups and two methyl groups. Invented by Russian chemist Aleksandr Dianin in 1891 and first synthesised by German chemist Theodor Zincke in 1905, BPA was shown to have oestrogenic properties in 1938, albeit weaker than those of estradiol-17B. Recent research has shown that BPA migrates from epoxy resins into food, sometimes reaching concentrations in excess of the European standard of 50 µg/kg.

The presence of BPA in many foods, particularly canned foods, raises public health concerns. Food is the main source human exposure to BPA, largely through canned foods. As an endocrine disruptor, BPA can interact with the receptors of oestrogens, and prolonged exposure to this compound can have adverse effects on health, influencing metabolism (type 2 diabetes, liver disorders, obesity), reproduction (sperm quality, sex hormone levels) and development (neurological and genital anomalies in children). Although numerous legal restrictions have been introduced in countries such as the European Union and the United States, BPA is still widely present in various everyday consumer products, particularly those that come into contact with food. This book offers a detailed analysis of the risks associated with the presence of BPA in our food and its direct impact on human health. Through an in-depth review of scientific research and global regulations, the book aims to raise awareness among both medical students and the general public of the public health issues raised by this chemical substance. By highlighting the effects of BPA on the human body and exploring possible alternatives, this book is an essential tool for understanding and reducing exposure to this endocrine disruptor.

ACKNOWLEDGEMENTS

I would like to express my deepest gratitude to my family, whose constant support and encouragement have been an invaluable source of motivation throughout writing of this book. To my parents, thank you for your unwavering love, wise counsel and unconditional support, which enabled me to overcome the challenges of this project. To my wife, thank you for your patience, understanding and strength, which have been essential in accompanying me on this intellectual adventure. And to my children, your enthusiasm and smiles have been a ray of sunshine, reminding me every day of the importance of sharing this knowledge for future generations. This book is as much yours as it is mine.

CONTENTS

1. GENERAL INFORMATION ON BISPHENOL A

The discovery of the ability of bisphenol A (BPA), a synthetic oestrogen, to migrate from epoxy resins and polycarbonate plastics into food has led to a worldwide mobilisation. This discovery triggered a series of studies aimed at understanding the factors influencing this migration, developing methods for measuring BPA in food matrices, assessing the level of human exposure, exploring less toxic alternatives, and introducing regulations to reduce the risks to people and the environment.

1.1. History

Bisphenol A was discovered in 1891 by the Russian chemist Aleksandr Dianin, then synthesised for the first time in 1905 by the German chemist Theodor Zincke. This compound is obtained by reacting two molecules of phenol with one molecule of acetone in the presence an acid catalyst. In the 1930s, BPA and other synthetic compounds were studied in the search for synthetic oestrogens for therapeutic use. However, because of its relatively low oestrogenic activity compared with that of estradiol, BPA was never used as a medicine. The pharmaceutical industry preferred another synthetic compound discovered at the same time, diethylstilbestrol, which showed stronger oestrogenic activity. In 1953, Dr Hermann Schnell, working for Bayer, succeeded in efficiently synthesising polycarbonate plastic by combining BPA with phosgene. From summer of 1960, the manufacture of BPA-based polycarbonate plastics expanded rapidly, reaching industrial production levels.

1.2. Definition and structure of BPA

Bisphenol A (see Figure 1), also known as 4,4'-isopropylidenediphenol and 2,2-bis(4-hydroxyphenyl)propane, is a solid, white synthetic compound with a faint phenolic odour. Its production is based on the reaction between one molecule acetone and two molecules of phenol. BPA is a xenoestrogen mainly used in the manufacture of epoxy resins and polycarbonate plastics. It can influence various biological processes and affect the metabolic, thyroid and androgenic systems.

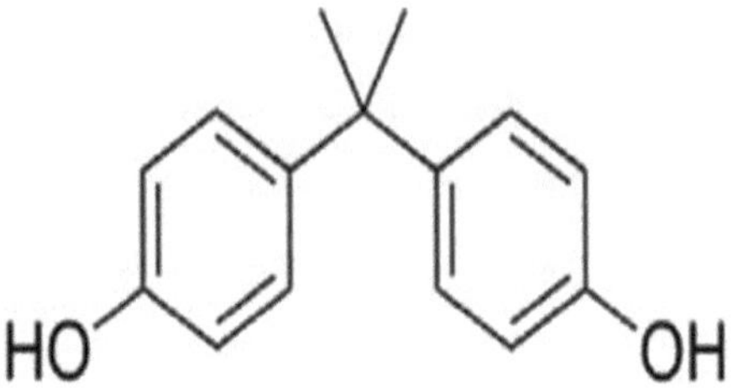

Figure 1: Structure of BPA.

1.3. Physico-chemical properties of BPA

1.3.1. Physical properties

Bisphenol A (BPA) is a white solid, available in crystals, powder or flakes. It is a small molecule with the molecular formula C1sH16O2 and a molecular weight of 228.29 g/mol. It has a density of 1.1 g/ml at 25°C, a melting point of between 158 and 159°C and a boiling point of around 250 to 252°C at a pressure of 1.7 kPa.BPA is highly soluble aqueous alkaline solutions, acetic acid and various organic solvents such as methanol, ethanol, acetonitrile and acetone. Its solubility in water is limited, at around 120 to 130 mg/L at 25°C, and it is also sparingly soluble in dichloromethane and very sparingly in n-heptane. Because of its With an n-octanol/water partition coefficient of 3.4, BPA is considered to be a relatively lipophilic substance.

Table 1: Physical properties of BPA.

Physical constants	Value
CAS No. (Chemical Abstracts Service registry number)	80-05-7
Molar mass	228.29 g/mol
Melting point	150°C to 157°C
Boiling point	360°C at 101.3 kPa 250 - 252°C at 1.7 kPa
Density	1.1 at 25°C
Vapour pressure	$5.3.10^{-9}$kPa at 25 °C 0.009 kPa at 190 °C
Flash	207 to 227°C
Auto-temperature inflammation	510 to 570 °C
Partition coefficient n-octanol/water	3,4

1.3.2. Chemical properties

BPA is stable under normal conditions, but slowly decomposes into phenol and isopropenylphenol at high temperatures. It exhibits pronounced exothermic reactivity with strong bases, chlorides and acid anhydrides, and can react violently with strong oxidants, posing fire and explosion hazards.

1.4. Industrial production and use

1.4.1. Industrial production

In 2012, global production of GAP exceeded 4.6 million tonnes. Asia produced more than half of this amount (53%), followed by Europe (25%) and North America (18%) (6). In 2015, around 7.7 million tonnes of BPA, worth $15.6 billion, were used in various industrial applications.

The global GAP market reached a value of $17.69 billion in 2017 and is expected to grow at an annual rate of 4.2% until 2026. The main consumers are China and other Asian countries, accounting for two-thirds of global consumption, followed by Europe and North and South America. These figures testify to a growing global demand for BPA, despite bans on its use in certain products intended for babies and young children.

1.4.2. Production processes

BPA (Figure 2) is produced by the condensation of two moles of phenol with one mole of acetone in the presence of an acid catalyst, such as hydrochloric acid, at a temperature of 60-80°C. This reaction can generate undesirable by-products, in particular BPA isomers and Dianin compound isomers. These impurities must be removed from the final product, for example by recrystallisation using chlorobenzene or aqueous alcohol, in order to obtain high-purity BPA.

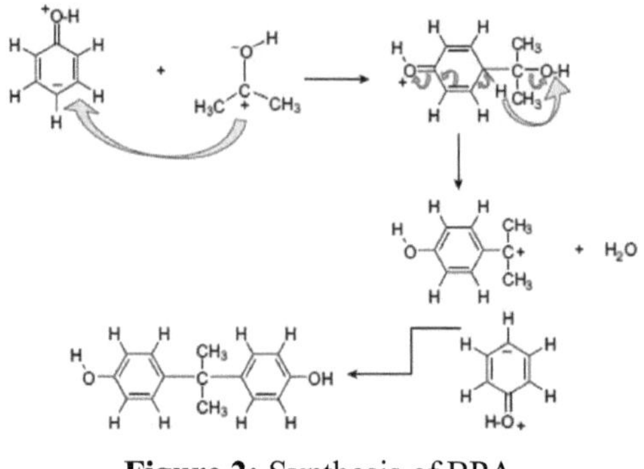

Figure 2: Synthesis of BPA.

BPA production processes have evolved over time. Conventional methods rely on a homogeneous liquid phase containing a strong acid, which requires corrosion-resistant materials and extensive facilities to recover the catalyst and purify the BPA. New approaches use a solid acid catalyst, often a sulphonic acid cation exchange resin. These resins offer excellent selectivity, reduce corrosion and enable high-quality BPA to be produced.

1.4.3. Use of BPA

BPA is an essential chemical molecule, mainly used in the manufacture of phenolic epoxy resins and polycarbonate plastics. It is also used to produce other polymers, such as polysulphone, polyacrylate and unsaturated polyester resins. These polymers have a wide range of applications, including thermal paper, food containers, flame retardants, medical devices, blood bags, construction materials, electronic components and automotive parts. In 2015, epoxy resins accounted for around 34% of global demand for BPA, mainly for the manufacture of surface coatings. Polycarbonate plastics accounted for 64% of demand, mainly supplying electronics, construction and automotive sectors. Demand for these polymers is expected to grow at an average annual rate of 3% for epoxy resins and 4% for polycarbonates.

- **Phenolic epoxy resins**

Epoxy resins, first synthesised by the Russian chemist Nikolai Prilezhaev, are low molecular weight molecules containing one or more of the following compounds functions epoxy functions FUNCTIONS (CH2OCH2). They are obtained by condensation of epichlorohydrin with BPA, in the presence a basic catalyst (Figure 3).

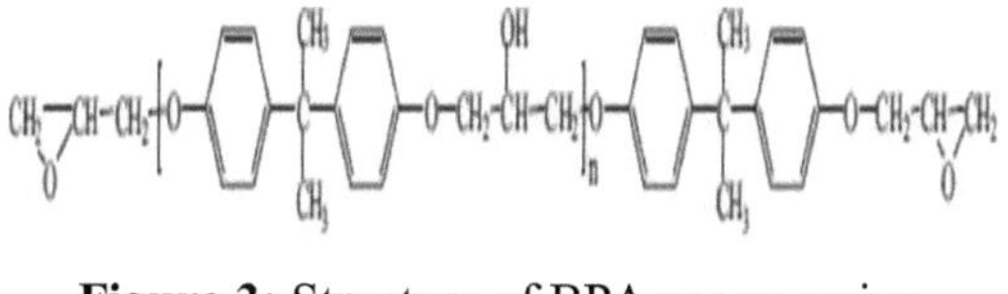

Figure 3: Structure of BPA epoxy resins.

BPA diglycidyl ether is the simplest form of BPA-based epoxy resins. The number repeating units in these resins influences their physical properties: low molecular weight molecules are generally liquids, while higher molecular weight molecules are viscous liquids or solids. Epoxy resins have many applications, particularly as interior coatings for metal containers. They offer protection against corrosion and prevent interaction between the container and its contents. Their effectiveness is based on several key properties: ease of handling, high safety, excellent resistance to solvents and chemicals, and impact resistance, low post-hardening shrinkage and excellent adhesion to a variety of substrates. Epoxy resins are also used in floor coverings, coatings, adhesives and sealants.

▶ Polycarbonate resins

Polycarbonate resins (Figure 4), which are macromolecular compounds, were traditionally produced using the phosgene ($COCl_2$) process, which is based on the interfacial polycondensation of BPA and $COCl_2$. However, this method has significant drawbacks linked to use of $COCl_2$, a highly toxic and corrosive reagent, and large quantities of methylene chloride as a solvent. To mitigate these impacts, more environmentally-friendly methods have been developed, such as the transesterification of BPA with diphenyl carbonate (DPC). Other options for the direct carbonisation of BPA use dimethyl carbonate (DMC) or carbon monoxide (CO) as alternative reagents.

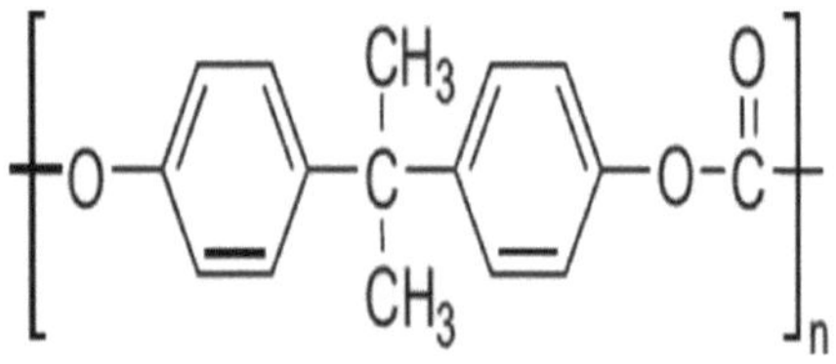

Figure 4: Structure of BPA polycarbonate resin.

Polycarbonate plastics are widely used in a variety of everyday objects, including plastic food containers, baby bottles, household appliance housings, safety glasses, hard hats, lenses, visors, as well as sockets, switches, bus shelters and lamp housings. These materials are preferred because of their many advantages over others plastics, such as their toughness, rigidity, transparency, physiological inertia and excellent thermal insulation properties.

2. CONTAMINATION OF THE ENVIRONMENT AND FOODSTUFFS BY THE BPA

2.1. Fate of BPA in the environment

BPA has been detected and quantified in various environmental samples, including indoor and outdoor air, sediments, agricultural soils, as well as lakes, rivers, oceans and groundwater. It has also been observed that concentrations of BPA in the environment vary seasonally, with higher levels in winter and lower levels in summer. Sediment is the most contaminated environment, due to its low oxygen content and high organic matter content, followed by water, soil finally air, where BPA concentrations are lowest.

The half-life of BPA in different environments is summarised in Table 2 below. BPA has a relatively long half-life in sediments, a shorter half-life water and soil, and a very short half-life in the atmosphere.

Table 2: Half-life of BPA in environmental matrices.

Matrix	Half-life in days
Atmosphere	0,13
Water	37,5
Soil	75
Sediment	337,5

The presence of oxygen plays an essential role in the degradation of BPA. When oxygen is present, BPA degrades rapidly and is not very persistent in the environment. In absence of oxygen, on the other hand, BPA is more stable, allowing it to remain in soil and water for a long time. Environmental contamination (Figure 5) results mainly from the discharge wastewater by industries manufacturing or using BPA as a raw material. Phytochemical degradation of products containing BPA also contributes to its dispersion. In this way, BPA can migrate through soil layers and seep into groundwater. Once in the aquatic environment, BPA can accumulate in the tissues of phytoplankton and microalgae, before contaminating other links in the food chain. This phenomenon exposes humans to BPA, mainly through the consumption of meat and other animal products.

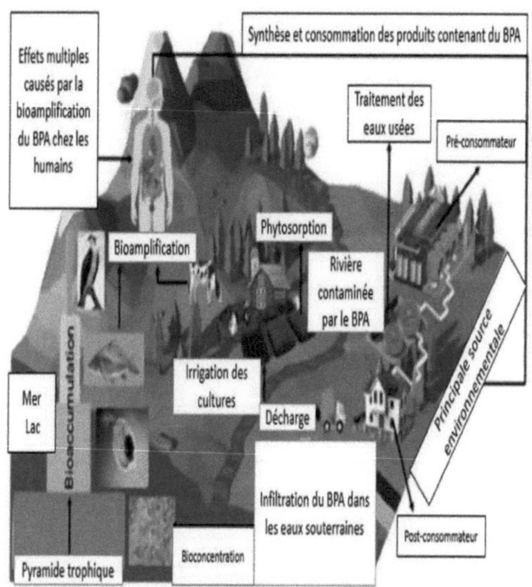

Figure 5: Fate of BPA in the environment.

2.2. Environmental contamination by BPA

The widespread use of products containing BPA, combined with inadequate processing methods and poor management of plastic waste, has led to the detection of this compound in various environmental media around the world.

2.2.1. Water

BPA, present in polycarbonate plastics and epoxy resins, is the main source of water contamination. Numerous studies carried out worldwide (Table 3) have assessed the presence of BPA in water, focusing particularly on rivers. Variable levels of BPA have been detected in water in different countries. For example, in China, BPA concentrations ranging from 23 to 195 ng/L have been found in urban river water in the Beijing-Tianjin-Hebei region. In the United States, BPA levels of between 50.3 and 74.4 ng/L have been measured in waste water. In Germany, India, Malaysia and South Africa, concentrations of BPA in river water have also been reported, ranging from 1.13 to 776 ng/L. In Iran, on the other hand, concentrations of BPA seawater are relatively low, not exceeding 16.71 ng/L.

Table 3: BPA levels in water.

Location	Type water	Concentration in ng/L
Germany	River water	8.9-776
India	River water	264-628
USA	Waste water	50.3-74.4
Iran	Coastal water	2.22-16.71
South Africa	River water	6,7-341,7
Malaysia	River water	1.13-5.52
China	Urban river water	23-195

The discharge of wastewater into rivers by industries that produce or recycle BPA-based materials is the main source of water pollution. Once in the environment, BPA can contaminate flora and fauna, cause health problems and lead to the death of children. This is a major ecological and health problem for the general population.

2.2.2. Air

The presence of BPA in air and dust (Table 4) has been reported in several studies. For example, a study conducted in Asia revealed BPA concentrations in urban air samples ranging from 30 to 17,400 pg/m3. BPA has also been detected in urban air in Spain, Vietnam, the United States and Malaysia, concentrations measured respectively at 108 pg/m^3, 1,050 to 11,200 pg/m^3, non-detectable at 137 pg/m^3 and 2,400 to 3,590 pg/m^3.In the United States, another study reported the detection of BPA in the air in industrial environments, with levels ranging from 0.010 to 920 pg/m^3, while in Malaysia, the concentrations observed in the industrial atmosphere ranged from 800 to 28,300 pg/m^3. The presence of BPA in the atmosphere is mainly due to poor combustion of materials containing BPA. This situation is particularly worrying in developing countries, where the incineration of domestic and industrial plastic waste is often unregulated and uncontrolled.

Table 4: Levels of BPA in air.

Location	Type air	Concentration in pg/m3
Beijing, China	Urban atmosphere	380-1260
Hong Kong	Urban atmosphere	30-690
Chennai, India	Urban atmosphere	200-17400
Sapporo, Japan	Urban atmosphere	70-930
In Corufia, Spain	Urban atmosphere	108 (Single sample)
Hanoi, Vietnam	Urban atmosphere	1050-11200
Minneapolis, USA	Urban atmosphere	ND-137
	Urban atmosphere	2400-3590
Malaysia	Industrial atmosphere	
	(Moulding plant of	800-28300
	plastic)	
	Industrial atmosphere	
	(Six companies	
USA	American manufacturers of	0.010-920
	BPA or products with	
	EPS basis)	

2.2. Contamination of consumer products and foodstuffs by BPA

2.2.1. Consumer products

BPA is present in a variety of everyday consumer products such thermal paper, personal care items, banknotes and plastic containers. A study conducted in the United States and China revealed that BPA was detected in a wide range of personal care products, with concentrations ranging from 0.35 to 44.3 µg/kg. This was confirmed by another study in China, where BPA was detected in 45.8% of the 150 personal care products examined, including sun creams, hand lotions, face masks and body lotions, with concentrations ranging from 12.8 to 168 µg/kg. BPA was also found in very low concentrations in feminine hygiene products. It is important to note that during the printing and colour development process on thermal paper, a large quantity of BPA is released onto its surface. Thermal paper can contain up to 42.6 g/kg of BPA.

2.2.2. Food

Although the assessment of BPA in fresh foods is not common, a few studies have indicated that it may be present in these products. BPA can enter the food chain at various stages of production, although the exact sources of contamination are still poorly understood. In France, one study detected BPA in meat and plant products at levels ranging from 0.105 to 82.73 µg/kg and 0.105 to 394.75 µg/kg respectively. Another study conducted three years later in the same country confirmed the presence of BPA in a wide range unpreserved foods of animal origin, at levels ranging from 0.09 to 60.1 µg/kg. In Spain, BPA was found in several unpreserved foods such as pâté, mushrooms, kidney beans, tuna and chicken. Canned foods, which are the main source human exposure BPA, relatively high concentrations due to migration of the substance from the lining of cans. Numerous studies around the world (Table 5) have reported the presence of BPA in canned foods, at varying levels, particularly in seafood, fruit and vegetables. In New Zealand, one study reported the detection of BPA in tuna, corned beef and coconut cream, with average concentrations of 109 µg/kg, 98 µg/kg and 191 µg/kg respectively. Another study reported the presence of BPA in various canned food products sold on the Canadian market, with average concentrations of 137 µg/kg for tuna, 105 µg/kg for condensed soups and 20 µg/kg for vegetables. These results have been confirmed by other studies carried out in France, the United States, the Netherlands, Spain, Nigeria and China. The highest concentrations of BPA have been detected in fish, particularly tuna. The leaching of microplastics into the aquatic environment may contribute to the direct contamination of fish by BPA.

Table 5: Levels of BPA in food.

Location Type food	µg/Kg
Tuna	109
New Zealand Corned of beef	98
Tuna	137
Vegetables	20
Vegetables	32.5
USA Fruit	0.4
Meat	1.5
Meat	9.71
Fish	11.9
Tuna	23
NetherlandsBas Viennese sausage	68
Tomato sauce	23
Beef corned beef	12.7
Nigeria Chicken	4.42
Fish	11.2
Tuna	32.22
Pâté	13.39
Spain Mushrooms	19.88
Chicken	20.91
Meat	77
Seafood products	47
China Fruit	60
Vegetables	18
Mushrooms	17
Average concentration in Canada France	

2.3. Regulations

The adverse effects of BPA on human health and the environment have prompted many countries to adopt restrictive measures aimed reducing exposure to this substance of concern, as shown in Figure 6.

2.3.1. Acceptable daily dose

The Acceptable Daily Intake (ADI) represents the maximum amount of BPA that can be consumed every day throughout a person's life, without causing any adverse effects on human health. In 2015the European Food Safety Authority (EFSA) established a temporary ADI (ADIt) for BPA of 4 µg/kg body weight (bw) per day, based on the toxic effects observed in laboratory animals, particularly on the kidneys and mammary glands. In 2023, following a request from the European Commission to re-evaluate this dose an EFSA expert group identified the immune system as the most vulnerable to BPA exposure. The study revealed that the critical effect of BPA was on Th17 cells in mice, leading to a reference point of 8.2 ng/kg bw per day, which was adjusted for humans. To establish the new ADI, an overall uncertainty of 50 was applied to take account of inter- and intra-species differences, resulting in a revised ADI of 0.2 ng/kg bw per day.Comparison of this new ADI of 0.2 ng/kg bw per day with estimates of average dietary exposure in Europe reveals that all population groups significantly exceed this limit. The average dietary intake of BPA is 875 ng/kg bw per day for infants and young children, 388 ng/kg bw per day for adults, and 1449 ng/kg bw per day for adolescents. This indicates that current dietary exposure to BPA in Europe constitutes a serious risk to public health. In the United States, the United States Food and Drug Administration (FDA) has set the ADI for BPA at 50 µg/kg bw, a limit that has remained unchanged since it was adopted in 2008.

2.3.2. Specific migration limit

The specific migration limit (SML) for BPA refers to the maximum quantity of this substance that can migrate from a packaging material to a food or food simulant. It is defined on the basis of the ADI and is intended to ensure that BPA does not pose a risk to human health when it comes into contact with food. In Europe, the SML for BPA has evolved over the years. It was 600 µg/kg food in 2011, when the ADI was set at 50 µg/kg bw. In 2018, this limit was reduced to 50 µg/kg, in correlation with a revised ADI of 4 µg/kg bw. With the new ADI of 0.2 ng/kg bw per day, it is expected that the SML for BPA will continue to decrease in the coming years.

2.3.3. Legal standards and restrictions

Faced with an increasing number of publications on the health risks of BPA and growing concerns about the safety of products in contact with polycarbonate plastics and epoxy resins, particularly infants and young children, several Western countries have taken steps to reduce exposure to this endocrine disruptor.In 2009, the Canadian government proposed an amendment to the Hazardous Products Act to include polycarbonate baby bottles containing BPA. This legislation came into force three years after the publication of EFSA's scientific opinion on BPA, which had established an ADI of 50 µg/kg body weight (bw) per day. It was also introduced a year after the FDA approved the same ADI. Canada has thus become the first country to regulate the use of BPA in materials in contact with foodstuffs. In 2011, the European Union adopted Regulation No. 10/2011, authorising the use of BPA as a monomer in plastics in contact with food, provided that the specific migration limit (SML) of BPA does not exceed 0.6 mg/kg of food. However, this regulation banned the use of products containing BPA in feeding bottles and packaging intended for infants and young children. In 2012, the FDA revised its regulations to ban the use of

BPA-based polycarbonate resins in baby bottles and sippy cups sold in the United States. A year later, this ban was extended to BPA-based epoxy resins used as coatings in infant formula packaging.In 2018, the EU published Regulation No. 213/2018, reducing the SML for BPA food to 50 µg/kg, following an EFSA expert opinion setting the temporary ADI for BPA at 4 µg/kg body weight per day. Then, in 2023, EFSA published a new expert report in which the ADI for BPA was re-evaluated and set at 0.2 ng/kg body weight per day, this new value representing the daily exposure threshold to avoid any health risk.However, in the countries Central and South America, as well in Africa and Asia, legislation has yet been adopted exposure to BPA, despite reports of BPA toxicity in food and surface water in these regions. It is now crucial to establish regulatory standards and legal limits for BPA in order to protect the health of people on these continents.

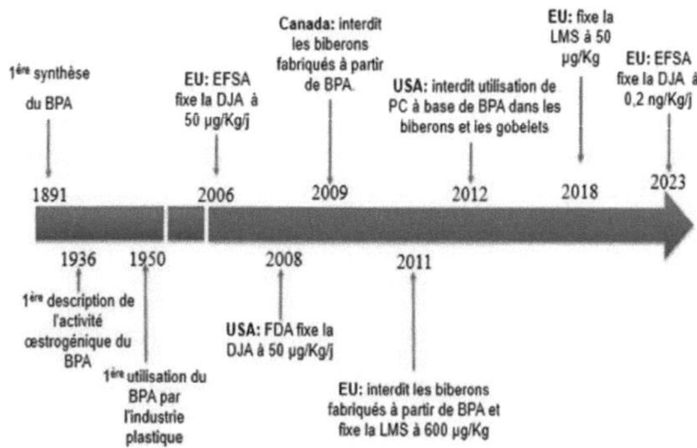

Figure 6: Evolution of BPA regulation around the world.

3. DOSAGE OF BPA

3.1. Factors influencing the migration of BPA in canned foods

The migration of BPA into canned foods can be influenced by a number of factors, including sterilisation temperature, storage time and food pH, each of which plays a crucial role in the amount of BPA transferred from packaging to food products.

3.1.1. Temperature

Temperature is a key factor in the release of BPA from cans. High temperatures encourage migration. For example, a study by Kawamura et al no significant migration of BPA at temperatures of 60 and 95°C 30 minutes' exposure. However, at 120°C, migration was notable, with BPA levels ranging from 35 to 124 µg/L. Other research, such as that by Krishnan et al, showed that heated water media in polycarbonate bottles induced elevated levels of progesterone receptors compared with media treated in autoclaved glass bottles, highlighting the impact of heat on BPA migration. In addition, the results of Munguia-Lopez et al. confirmed that high-temperature heat treatment promotes BPA migration.

3.1.2. Contact time

The length of contact between food and the lining of cans is also a key factor in BPA migration. Several studies have found that the longer the contact time, the greater the amount of BPA migrated. Cao et al, for example, found that nine infant food showed additional BPA migration after 10 months' storage at room temperature, with migration increases ranging from 29.8% to 110%. However, Munguia-Lopez et al. reported results of contradictory, observing that no effect of storage time was noted BPA migration in cans of tuna, while an effect was observed in cans of jalapenos. In addition, Biles et al. noted that BPA migration was higher in cans agitated by a blender than in those left in static conditions.

3.1.3. pH of food

The pH of canned foods has an impact on BPA migration, although the results of studies are sometimes contradictory. Some research suggests that an increase in pH leads to an increase in the release of BPA. Benhamada et al. confirmed that increasing pH promotes BPA release, while Biedermann-Brem et al. found that a 3% citric acid solution significantly reduced BPA release by up to 10-fold. Conversely, Yonekibo et al. found that there was no significant correlation between pH and BPA levels in canned foods. In contrast, Munguia-Lopez et al. found high levels of BPA migration (65.45 μg/L) in 3% acetic acid (pH below 4.5) after heating at 121°C for 90 minutes. Their study concluded that lowering the pH significantly increased the release of BPA.

3.1.4. Lipid content of foods

BPA, being a lipophilic chemical, tends to concentrate more fat-rich foods. This characteristic is responsible for the high concentrations of BPA observed in products such as infant milk. According to a study by Santillana et al, the level of BPA migration in infant formula was higher than in food simulants such 50% ethanol and acetic acid. Similarly, Johnson et al. reported that the level of BPA migration in milk was slightly higher than the levels observed in water and apple juice. In addition to fat content, a number of other factors can also affect BPA levels in canned foods. These include the methods used to manufacture the , the type food (salty, sweet or high-fat), the mineral composition of the food and the repeated use or ageing of the cans.

3.2. Determination of BPA in food matrices

Improved analytical techniques are essential for detecting toxic compounds present at extremely low concentrations in food products. The ability to detect these low concentrations in complex food samples has become a priority in recent scientific advances. This is driven by the need ensure maximum precision in the determination of these trace substances, which is a major challenge for current analytical methods. The process of preparing food samples for BPA analysis (Figure 7) follows a number of conventional steps, including pre-treatment, extraction and instrumental analysis.

3.2.1. Sample pre-treatment

Sample pre-treatment is a key step in ensuring the sensitivity and selectivity required for accurate BPA analysis. For solid foods, this stage generally begins with homogenisation to standardise the composition of the sample, making it easier to handle and process in the laboratory. Once homogenised, the samples allow a uniform distribution of constituents, which is crucial for obtaining reliable results. In the case of liquid foods, they are often filtered to separate any solid particles or impurities that might interfere with the analysis, thus ensuring the purity of the sample. Sometimes additional steps are required for certain types food specific requirements. For example, in the case of carbonated drinks, the elimination of air can be essential proceeding with the analysis. In addition, for protein-rich samples, a protein precipitation step is often required to remove the proteins, thus ensuring greater precision in the analytical results. In short, sample pre-treatment is a crucial stage that requires particular attention to ensure the validity and quality of the results obtained subsequent analysis.

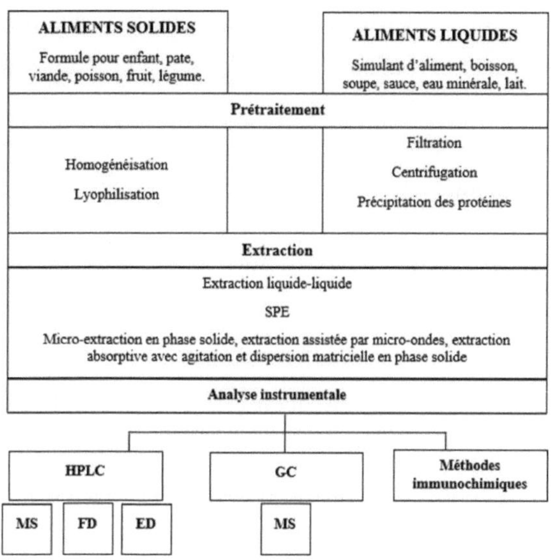

Figure 7: General diagram of BPA analysis in food.

3.2.2. Extraction

The isolation of BPA from food samples is mainly carried by solvent extraction and solid phase extraction (SPE) methods, which are widely preferred because of their simplicity and flexibility. The solvent evaporation step, carried out after extraction, is necessary because of the low concentration of BPA in food samples. In solvent extraction, also known as liquid-liquid extraction, various solvents can be used, either alone or in a mixture. Acetonitrile is the most commonly used solvent. It has been used to extract BPA from a variety of products, such as vegetable oils, PVC films, vegetables, fruit, fish, soups, fatty food simulants and canned foods in oily, aqueous or acidic media. It has also been used to extract BPA from canned pet food. In addition, methanol-water and ethanol-water mixtures have been used extract BPA from infant milk powders, while dichloromethane has been used to extract BPA from soft drinks. Solid phase extraction generally uses a vacuum manifold for SPE, a vacuum pump and specific extraction columns containing Florisil or silica gel. Other methods, although less commonly used, have been applied for the extraction of BPA, such as solid-phase microextractionmicrowave-assisted extraction, absorptive extraction with stirring and solid-phase matrix dispersion.

3.2.3. Instrumental analysis

The separation, identification and quantification of BPA are reliably achieved using chromatographic techniques such as high performance liquid chromatography (HPLC) and gas chromatography (GC). The most common chromatographic methods for determining BPA include HPLC coupled to a fluorescence detector (FD) or to mass spectrometry (MS), as well as GC. gas chromatography coupled with mass spectrometry (GC-MS). For example, Braunrath et al. used high-performance liquid chromatography with fluorescence detection (HPLC/FD) to identify BPA in various food matrices. Their study revealed variable recovery rates of BPA, depending the specific composition each food. In another study, Li et al. detected and quantified BPA in soft drinks using the HPLC/FD method, with limits of quantification of between 0.06 and 0.1 µg/L. Vilarinho et al. also quantified BPA in canned vegetables using the HPLC/FD method, with detection and quantification limits of 5 µg/kg and 10 µg/kg respectively.

4. TOXIC EFFECTS OF BPA

4.1. Human exposure to BPA

4.1.1. Exposure to BPA food

Food is the main source human exposure to BPA, with exposure levels generally at least ten times higher than those from other non-food sources, for all age . EFSA, in an opinion published in 2015, confirmed that food is the main source of exposure to BPA, with canned foods playing a major role in this exposure. In Europe, the average dietary intake of BPA was estimated at 875 ng/kg body weight per day for infants and young children, 388 ng/kg body weight per day for adults and 1449 ng/kg body weight per day for adolescents. In the United States, dietary exposure to BPA was estimated at 12.6 ng/kg body weight per day, of which 12.4 ng/kg body weight came from canned foods. In China, total dietary exposure to BPA was estimated at 55.2 ng/kg body weight per day, while that from canned foods 32.9 ng/kg body weight per day. These figures show that in most countriesdaily dietary exposure to BPA far exceeds the new acceptable daily intake set by EFSA for 2023 at 0.2 ng/kg body weight per day.

4.1.2. Occupational exposure to BPA

Workers in industries producing or processing BPA may be exposed to this substance via the dermal or respiratory route. A study carried out in the United States revealed that the total urinary concentration of BPA in workers in the industries concerned was 88.0 µg/g, almost 70 times higher than that of American adults (1.27 µg/g). A study in Malaysia found that workers in a injection moulding workers had an average concentration of BPA in their urine of 3.81 ng/ml, much higher than that of control subjects (0.73 ng/ml). Moreover, this concentration was significantly correlated with the level of BPA in the air.

In some countries, regulatory measures have been introduced to limit occupational exposure to BPA. In the EU, for example, the maximum level of BPA in inhalable dust in industrial environments is set at 2 mg/m^3.

4.1.3. Other sources exposure to BPA

There are several other sources contributing to the overall exposure of the population to BPA:

- **Inhalation of dust**: Average exposure in the EU is 0.6 ng/kg body weight per day in adults and 8.8 ng/kg body weight per day in children.
- **Dermal exposure to thermal paper**: In Europe, average exposure levels are 58.9 ng/kg body weight per day in adults.
- **Dermal exposure to cosmetic products**: Exposure levels vary from 2 ng/kg body weight per day in adults to 4.8 ng/kg body weight per day in children.
- **Chewing toys**: Average exposure values in Europe range from 0.01 to 0.2 ng/kg body weight per day in children.

4.2. Toxicity of BPA

4.2.1. Toxicokinetics of BPA

Oral and dermal exposure to BPA leads to rapid and significant absorption. Once in the body, BPA diffuses into tissues, crosses the placental barrier and is detected in breast milk. The majority of BPA metabolites are eliminated in the urine, with less than 10% in the form of unchanged BPA.

▶ **Absorption**

The main exposure to this substance in humans is via the oral route. In one study, 100 µg/kg body weight of deuterium BPA (d6-BPA), a stable isotope of BPA, was administered to a group of men and women in biscuits. The BPA was rapidly absorbed from the digestive tract and detected in the serum only five minutes after administration. Almost all of the BPA administered (84-109%) was found in the urine, and the majority of participants excreted 90% of the BPA metabolites within 24 hours.For dermal exposure, in another study after application of d6-BPA at a dose of 100 µg/kg for 12 hours to 10 subjects, 2.2% of the dermally applied dose reached the general circulation. BPA was detected in serum 1.4 hours after application.

▶ Distribution

The distribution of BPA in the body depends on its passage from the blood to the tissues. A study of six mammalian species estimated that the volume of distribution of BPA will vary according to species, ranging from 0.44 L/kg in mice to 231.9 L/kg in horses. For a 70 kg man, this represents an estimated volume of distribution of 69.67 L. BPA is distributed mainly to tissues and fat, and is mainly bound to plasma proteins, particular albumin and SHBG (Sex Hormone-Binding Globulin), with around 95% of BPA bound to proteins and only 5% remaining in free form.

▶ Oral bioavailability

The oral bioavailability of BPA is low due to its intense metabolism in the liver. In rats, mice and monkeys, the bioavailability of unconjugated BPA is estimated at 2.8%, 0.45% and 0.9% respectively, taking into account the hepatic first-pass effect. Although BPA is completely absorbed from the gastrointestinal tract, the low bioavailability is due to its degradation in the liver before reaching the systemic circulation.

▶ Metabolism

BPA metabolism involves phase I and II reactions that transform BPA into more hydrophilic metabolites, facilitating its elimination via the urine. Free BPA represents less than 1% of the total BPA excreted in urine and blood. The main metabolite of BPA is BPA-glucuronide (BPA-G), formed by the addition of glucuronic acid by enzyme UGT (uridine 5'-diphospho-glucuronosyltransferase) in the liver, and eliminated in the urine.

BPA sulphate (BPA-S) is another major metabolite of BPA, although its formation is only a secondary pathway. BPA is mainly excreted as BPA-G (94.6%), with only traces of BPA-S and free BPA (3.7% and 1.7%, respectively). Phase I reactions, catalysed by cytochrome P450 enzymes, generate hydroxylated metabolites such as ortho-hydroxylated BPA, which can react with GSH to form reactive conjugates. Other metabolites such as MBP (4-methyl-2,4-bis(4-hydroxyphenyl)pent-1-ene) and IPP (isopropenylphenol) are also produced and have a much more potent oestrogenic activity than BPA, being 500 and 100 times stronger respectively. However, BPA-G and BPA-S did not show any oestrogenic activity.

Figure 8 illustrates the different metabolic pathways of BPA.

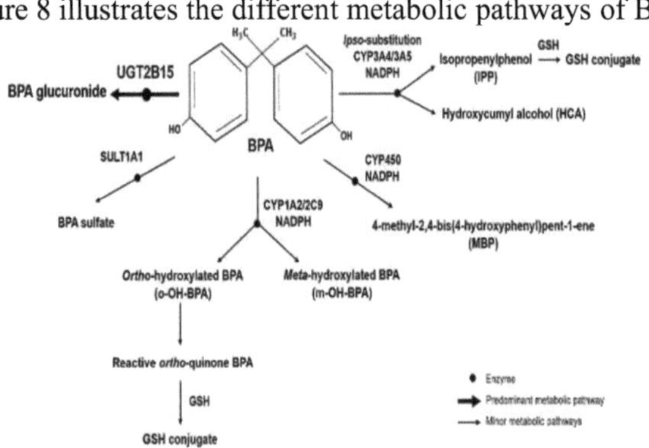

Figure 8: Metabolic pathways of BPA.

- **Elimination**

BPA is rapidly absorbed from the digestive tract after ingestion and metabolised by the liver into water-soluble conjugates. These conjugates are almost entirely eliminated in the urine in humans and in the faeces in animals. In an experimental study, the plasma clearance (Cl) and half-life (t1/2) of BPA were calculated after intravenous administration of BPA to six mammalian species. The results obtained in animals were used to estimate Cl and t1/2 in humans at 1.79 L/min and 2.29 h, respectively. Another human study estimated the Cl and t1/2 of BPA to be 1.6 L/min and 6.4 h, respectively. This study reported that BPA is completely eliminated in the urine 24 hours after ingestion, mainly in the form of BPA-G (87%) and BPA-S (), while free BPA represents only 0.11% of the forms eliminated in the urine.

- **Mechanism of action**

BPA can accumulate in various tissues and organs and be harmful to human health through a variety of molecular mechanisms. BPA can bind to oestrogen receptors a and B and have an impact on body weight and tumorigenesis by interfering with oestrogen receptor (ER) signalling. The affinity of BPA for ERB receptors is 6 to 10 times greater than for ERa receptors, while its affinity for oestrogen receptors is much lower than that of estradiol. What's more, it can also bind with high affinity to receptors gamma linked to oestrogens.BPA can bind to many other nuclear receptors, such as GPR30, and affect cancer metabolism and progression, androgen receptors and disrupt male reproductive capacity, thyroid hormone receptors and T3 activity or disrupt thyroid function, as well as glucocorticoid receptors (GR) with a lower intensity than cortisol, exerting a synergistic effect on adipogenesis. Several transcription factors are involved in the toxic action of BPA on fat and liver homeostasis (obesogenic effect), the cardiovascular system and cancer. Finally, BPA causes epigenetic changes, such as histone modification, changes in microRNA expression and DNA methylation.

4.2. Toxic effects of BPA on humans

The development of pathologies results a combination of genetic and environmental factors, and exposure to xenobiotics has been suggested as a contributor to these pathological processes. Chronic exposure to BPA may be responsible for adverse effects on reproduction, metabolism, development and immunity.

▶ Reproduction and fertility

BPA can alter sperm quality, reproductive hormones and couples' fertility. Li et al have demonstrated the existence of a negative correlation between urinary BPA levels and the quality of sperm parameters. An increase in the level BPA in the urine is linked to a decrease in the concentration and total number of spermatozoa, their vitality and motility. In addition, Zhou et al. found that high serum levels of BPA increase levels of sex hormone-binding globulin and reduce levels of free testosterone, androstenedione and the the of androgens index. Ehrlich et al. examined the success rate implantation in women undergoing in vitro fertilisation and found that those with highest concentrations of BPA had twice the risk of implantation failure. Similarly, Bloom et al. evaluated the embryo fragmentation score and the number of embryonic cells during in vitro fertilisation and found that high serum levels of BPA in men can affect embryo quality. A study by Tarantino et al measured serum BPA in women with polycystic ovary syndrome (PCOS) and in controls. The results showed that women with PCOS had significantly higher serum BPA levels than controls. Increased spleen size was also associated with higher BPA levels.

Finally, Itoh et al. measured urinary BPA in infertile women diagnosed with endometriosis, observing a positive correlation between urinary BPA levels and the most severe forms of this pathology. However, this correlation became insignificant after adjustment for urinary creatinine.

▶ Development

Numerous recent epidemiological studies have highlighted negative impact of prenatal or pre-pubertal exposure on children's development. Prenatal exposure to BPA can alter children's birth weight. One study conducted by Miao et al. demonstrated a linear dose-response relationship between prenatal exposure to BPA and lower birth weight. Children born to exposed mothers had significantly lower birth weights than children whose mothers were exposed to BPA. Whose the mothers were not exposed. BPA can also disrupt children's neurological behaviour, causing hyperactivity and aggression. Braun et al measured urinary BPA levels in pregnant women at 16 and 24 weeks' gestation, as well as at the time of delivery. When the children reached the age of 2, their behaviour was assessed. A significant correlation was observed between higher levels of maternal BPA and an increase in hyperactivity and aggression in the girls. In contrast, no relationship was observed in boys. This study revealed that the :S 16-week gestation period could be a critical phase of prenatal exposure to BPA. In addition, Perera et al found a correlation between urinary BPA levels at 34 weeks' and behavioural problems in children aged between 3 and 5 years. Boys showed high scores in emotional reactivity and aggressive behaviour, while girls showed lower scores in all categories. BPA can also cause male genital abnormalities, in particular a reduction in ano-genital distance. One study found a correlation between prenatal exposure to BPA and reduced ano-genital distance in boys whose mothers had been occupationally exposed to BPA. However, no correlation was found with cryptorchidism.

▶ Metabolism

Numerous human studies have established a link between BPA and cardiovascular disease, liver disease, abnormal thyroid function and type 2 diabetes. High levels of urinary BPA were closely linked to a higher probability of diagnosis of cardiovascular diseases, such angina pectoris, myocardial infarction, heart attacks and peripheral arterial disease in adults. Melzer et al. followed individuals with and controls for 10.8 years, and found that higher concentrations of urinary BPA were positively associated with a higher incidence of coronary heart disease. Olsen et al. reported a significant correlation between elevated serum BPA concentrations and increased levels of low-density and high-density lipoproteins in individuals aged 70. They also found less pronounced links with the coronary heart disease. Exposure to BPA has also been associated with the development of type 2 diabetes. Lang et al observed a strong association between type 2 diabetes and high levels of urinary BPA. However, blood glucose levels measured in the same patients were not significantly correlated with BPA concentrations, suggesting that diabetes drugs may alter blood glucose levels and mask the correlation with type 2 diabetes. Silver et al. also observed a significant association between high levels of urinary BPA and an increased risk of type 2 diabetes, as well as an increase in HbA1c levels in the blood. Chronic exposure to BPA can influence thyroid function humans. Wang et al. studied workers occupationally exposed to BPA and observed a correlation between elevated levels of BPA in the urine and increased levels of free T3 in the blood. In addition, Chevrier et al. monitored urinary BPA concentrations in pregnant mothers on several occasions during pregnancy and found a significant association between high maternal BPA levels and low T4 levels. Maternal BPA was negatively related to neonatal TSH in boys, but no association was was observed in the girls. Finally, Brucker-Davis al. monitored mothers and their newborns by analysing BPA levels in materrial serum and found a negative correlation between BPA and TSH in the newborns.

▶ Immunity

Exposure to BPA during childhood development can lead to immunomodulation and the development of diseases such as allergy, asthma, multiple sclerosis and type 1 diabetes. BPA can modulate immune function through various processes, such as agonist and antagonist effects on several receptors, epigenetic modifications, as well by disrupting cell signalling pathways and the intestinal microbiome. This leads to a reduction in regulatory T cells, an increase in pro- and anti-inflammatory cytokines, and altered function of the innate and adaptive immune systems.

▶ Hormone-dependent cancer

Various xenoestrogens, including BPA, are suspected of playing a role in the development of cancer. Janet et al. studied the response of prostate cancer cells to exposure to BPA and dihydrotestosterone (DHT). They found that BPA and DHT distinct gene responses, significantly reducing the expression of the oestrogen receptor beta. BPA may therefore specifically stimulate the proliferation of prostate tumour cells. Morgan et al. studied urinary BPA levels in women with gynaecological cancer and found higher levels of BPA in those with ovarian cancer. However, no significant association was found between BPA and gynaecological cancers. However, cross-sectional epidemiological studies have several limitations that likely to introduce bias into their results. Overall, these studies do not provide solid, consistent evidence establishing an association between exposure to BPA and the development of different types of cancer.

5. ANALOGUES OF BPA

In recent years, a great deal of research has been devoted to finding alternatives to BPA, due to health concerns linked to its use in materials in contact with food and the restrictions imposed by regulations on packaging for certain . All in all, 16 BPA analogues have been used to replace BPA in various industrial applications. Of these, three main analogues dominate the market: GMP (4,4'-methylene diphenyl), BPS (bis(4-hydroxyphenyl)sulphone) and BPAF (2,2-bis(4-hydroxyphenyl)hexafluoropropylene).

Products containing these alternatives to BPA are often labelled "BPA-free". However, this may wrongly lead people to believe that these products are safe, whereas the safety of BPA analogues remains largely unexplored. In the past, BPA was the most frequently detected bisphenol in environmental monitoring studies. Today, GMP and BPS are also commonly identified, and high concentrations of GMP, BPS and BPAF have been found in water, air, soil and even human body fluids. In addition, BPA analogues are present in everyday consumer articles, and several of these compounds present health impacts or toxic effects at concentration levels comparable to or even lower than those of BPA.

5.1. Contamination de l'environnement par les analogues de BPA The structural analogues of BPA identified and quantified in the environment include BPAF, BPAP, BPB, BPF, BPP, BPS and BPZ . Liao et al. measured the concentration of eight bisphenols in sediments collected from various industrialised areas the United States, Japan and Korea. The total concentration of bisphenols detected (BPA, BPAF, BPS, BPAP, BPF) in sediments ranged from < LQ to 25.3 µg/g dry weight, with a mean value of 0.201 µg/g dry weight. In addition, Song et al. measured the concentrations BPA analogues in sludge collected from 52 municipal wastewater plants in China, and the concentrations of BPA analogues in the sediments of these plants. The mean concentrations detected were 3.84, 3.02 and 4.69 ng/g for GMP, BPS and BPAF, respectively. In another study by Yamazaki et al, the concentrations of eight BPA analogues, including BPS and BPF, were measured in surface water taken from various rivers in Japan, Korea, China and India. The concentrations found ranged from ND to 277 ng/L for GMP and from ND to 26.5 ng/L for BPS.

5.2. Food contamination by analogues of BPA

BPA analogues have been detected in various food categories, with concentrations varying according to the type food and the country origin. A study carried out in Italy by Grumetto et al examined the presence of BPB in canned tomatoes of various brands purchased in Italian supermarkets. Of the 42 samples analysedBPB was detected in 9, with concentrations ranging from 27.1 to 85.7 µg/kg. Another study conducted in the United States revealed the presence of BPA analogues in 75% of the 267 food samples tested. Average concentrations were 3 µg/kg for BPA, 0.01 µg/kg for BPAF, 0.06 µg/kg for BPAP, 0.01 µg/kg for BPB, 0.93 µg/kg for BPF, 0.21 µg/kg for BPP, 0.16 µg/kg for BPS, 0.03 µg/kg for BPZ and 0.21 µg/kg for BPP. In addition, a study conducted in Spain reported the presence of BPS in canned foods, with concentrations ranging from ND to 36.1 µg/kg.

5.3. Human exposure to BPA analogues

Recent studies have shown the presence of several BPA analogues in biological fluids. Asimakopoulos et al analysed eight bisphenols (BPA, BPAS, BPAF, BPB, BPAP, BPP, BPZ and BPF) in 130 urine samples collected from the population of the city of Jeddah, Saudi Arabia. All the bisphenols were present in the urine, but their concentrations varied considerably, with mean concentrations ranging from 0.16 µg/L for BPZ and BPB to 13.3 µg/L for BPS. Concentrations of BPS were higher than those of BPA, with detection rates of 100% and 86.2% respectively. Another study conducted in China measured the levels of 13 bisphenols in the urine samples of 42 children. Total urinary concentrations of bisphenols ranged from 0.38 to 24.45 μg/L, with a median of 2.08 μg/L. BPA and BPS were detected in over 98% of samples, while GMP and BPE were present in 28% and 26% of samples, respectively. The other bisphenols were not detected. A study conducted in Poland assessed serum levels of BPA, BPS and GMP in 199 women with polycystic ovary syndrome (PCOS) and 158 controls. BPA and BPS were detected in 95% of samples, GMP was detected in 71%. Mean concentrations 0.39 μg/L, 0.12 μg/L and 0.10 μg/L respectively. In women with PCOS, serum BPS levels were significantly higher than in controls, while BPA and GMP levels were not significantly different.

5.4. Toxicity of BPA analogues

Data on the potential toxic effect of BPA structural analogues on human health is limited, or even non-existent for some of them. Available research has identified a range of toxic effects associated with these analogues, including endocrine disruption, reproductive toxicity, cytotoxicity, genotoxicity, neurotoxic effects and dioxin-like effects. BPS and GMP have similar hormonal activity to BPA, particularly in terms of oestrogenic, anti-oestrogenic, androgenic and anti-androgenic activity, both in vitro and in vivo. In addition, BPS acts in a similar way to estradiol in membrane-mediated pathways, which are crucial for cellular processes such as proliferation, differentiation and apoptosis. For other BPA analogues, such as BPAF, BPE, BPM and BPZ, the available data suggest a risk of reproductive toxicity with a possible mechanism action as endocrine disruptors. However, for BPC, BPAP and BPP, the possible toxic effects on health have not yet been explored.

6. RECOMMENDATIONS

In view of the risks associated with exposure to BPA for individual and collective health, we propose the following recommendations aimed at reducing this exposure, particularly in developing countries.

Recommendations for leaders of developing countries :

- **Set strict limits** on the migration of BPA into foodstuffs in contact with polycarbonate plastics and epoxy resins, to guarantee food safety.
- **Banning the use of BPA** in packaging for infant and toddler formula, in particular polycarbonate plastics and epoxy resins, which represent an increased health risk for the most vulnerable.
- **Reinforce the management waste containing BPA**, by prohibiting its dumping or uncontrolled incineration, to limit environmental pollution and protect public health.
- **Set up approved centres** to carry out regular checks BPA levels in food products, thus ensuring ongoing quality monitoring.
- **Encourage industry** to adopt less toxic alternatives to BPA, by providing incentives for research and the use of safe materials. In addition, manufacturers should be required to provide full and clear information on packaging, particularly on the pH of products.
- **Promote safe alternatives**, such as glass bottles, for acidic and fatty food products, to reduce consumer exposure to the risks of BPA.
- **Limit the shelf life of canned products** to one year from the date of manufacture, in order to reduce the risks associated with the deterioration of packaging materials and the migration of BPA.
- **Conduct awareness campaigns** to inform the public about the dangers of BPA, particularly for children and pregnant women, and to encourage safer

consumption behaviour.

Recommendations for consumers :

- **Encourage the consumption fresh food** whenever possible, in order to exposure to chemicals in packaging.
- **Choose products with BPA-free packaging**, to limit the risks associated with this substance.
- **Avoid heating food in cans** in their original packaging, as this can encourage BPA migration. In the event of prolonged storage, it is preferable to transfer food to BPA-free glass or plastic containers.
- **Do not buy canned food with** a manufacturing date older than 12 months, to ensure that the packaging materials have not been altered by time, which can increase the migration of BPA.

CONCLUSION

At the end of this , it is clear that Bisphenol A (BPA) is a silent threat, omnipresent in our daily lives. Its presence in our food and everyday products raises essential questions about public health and the need to take measures to limit our exposure to this substance.

As a society, we have a duty to protect future generations from the potentially serious effects of BPA. Scientific progress and increased awareness are opening up the prospect of solutions and alternatives, but there is still a great deal to be done, both in terms of public policy and individual behaviour. This book not only takes stock of the current situation, it is also a call for collective action.

For medical students, researchers and health professionals, it is essential to incorporate the issues surrounding chemical pollution into our practices and therapeutic strategies. For the general public, greater awareness of the impact of our consumer choices on health and the environment can trigger positive change.

So this book, born of deep passion and sincere commitment, represents a first step towards a future where informed decisions and prevention will guide our actions to preserve public health and improve quality of life. It is not a definitive conclusion, but a starting point for ongoing reflection and action.

BIBLIOGRAPHY

1. Featherstone S. A Complete Course in Canning and Related Processes: Volume 3 Processing Procedures for Canned Food Products. 14th Edition. Sawston: Woodhead Publishing; 2015.

2. Allard P. bisphenol A. In: Gupta RC. Biomarkers in toxicology. 1st Edition. Boston: Academic Press; 2014.p. 459-474.

3. Ineris. Technical and economic data on chemical substances in France: Bisphenol A. 2010. p. 77.

4. Dodds EC, Lawson W. Molecular structure in relation to oestrogenic activity. Compounds without a phenanthrene nucleus. Proceedings of the Royal Society of London Series B-Biological Sciences. 1938;125(839):222-232.

5. Vilarinho F, Sendón R, Van der Kellen A, Vaz M, Silva AS. Bisphenol A in food as a result of its migration from food packaging. Trends in food science & technology. 2019;91:33-65.

6. Russo G, Barbato F, Mita DG, Grumetto L. Occurrence of Bisphenol A and its analogues in some foodstuff marketed in Europe. Food and Chemical Toxicology. 2019;131:110575.

7. Commission Regulation (EU) 2018/213 of 12 February 2018 on the use of bisphenol A in varnishes and coatings intended to come into contact with food and amending Regulation (EU) No 10/2011 as regards the use of this substance in plastic food materials, (2018).

8. Fan AM, Chou W-C, Lin P. Toxicity and risk assessment of bisphenol A. In: Gupta RC. Reproductive and Developmental Toxicology. 3rd Edition. Boston: Academic Press; 2017. p. 765-795.

9. Lorber M, Schecter A, Paepke O, Shropshire W, Christensen K, Birnbaum L. Exposure assessment of adult intake of bisphenol A (BPA) with emphasis on canned food dietary exposures. Environment international. 2015;77:55-62.

10. Kitamura S, Suzuki T, Sanoh S, Kohta R, Jinno N, Sugihara K, et al. Comparative study of the endocrine- disrupting activity of bisphenol A and 19 related compounds. Toxicological Sciences. 2005;84(2):249-259.
11. Rochester JR. Bisphenol A and human health: a review of the literature. Reproductive toxicology. 2013;42:132- 155.
12. Krishnan AV, Stathis P, Permuth SF, Tokes L, Feldman D. Bisphenol-A: an estrogenic substance is released from polycarbonate flasks during autoclaving. Endocrinology. 1993;132(6):2279-2286.
13. Dodds EC, Goldberg L, Lawson W, Robinson R. Oestrogenic activity of certain synthetic compounds. Nature. 1938;141(3562):247-248.
14. INRS. Bisphenol A: Fiche toxicologique n°279. 2022. p. 16.
15. Miyagawa S, Sato T, Iguchi T. Bisphenol A. In: Ando H, Ukena K, Nagata S. Handbook of Hormones. 2nd Edition. San Diego: Academic Press; 2021. p. 1003-1004.
16. Xiao C, Wang L, Zhou Q, Huang X. Hazards of bisphenol A (BPA) exposure: A systematic review of plant toxicology studies. Journal of hazardous materials. 2020;384:121488.
17. Almeida S, Raposo A, Almeida-Gonzalez M, Carrascosa C. Bisphenol A: Food exposure and impact on human health. Comprehensive reviews in food science and food safety. 2018;17(6):1503-1517.
18. Torres-García JL, Ahuactzin-Pérez M, Fernández FJ, Cortés-Espinosa DV. Bisphenol A in the environment and recent advances in biodegradation by fungi. Chemosphere. 2022;303:134940.
19. Markit I. Bisphenol A: Chemical economics handbook. 2022; Available at: https://www.spglobal.com/commodityinsights/en/ci/products/bisphenol-chemical-economics-handbook.html.
20. Kyriacos D. Polycarbonates. In: Gilbert M. Brydson's Plastics Materials. 8th Edition: Butterworth- Heinemann; 2017. p. 457-485.
21. Gálvez-Ontiveros Y, Moscoso-Ruiz I, Rodrigo L, Aguilera M, Rivas A,

Zafra-Gómez A. Presence of parabens and bisphenols in food commonly consumed in Spain. Foods. 2021;10(1):92.
22. Badding MA, Vargas JR, Fortney J, Cheng QJ, Ho C-H. Toxicological risk assessment of bisphenol a released from dialyzers under simulated-use and exaggerated extraction conditions. Regulatory Toxicology and Pharmacology. 2020;118:104787.
23. McCann SR. Plastic in blood and wine. Bone Marrow Transplantation. 2021;56(4):762-764.
24. May C. Epoxy resins: chemistry and technology. New York: Routledge; 2018.
25. Nicolais L, Borzacchiello A, Lee SM. Wiley encyclopedia of composites. 2nd Edition: Wiley Online Library; 2012. 3444 p.
26. Jin F-L, Li X, Park S-J. Synthesis and application of epoxy resins: A review. Journal of Industrial and Engineering Chemistry. 2015;29:1-11.
27. Jin FL, Park SJ. Thermal properties and toughness performance of hyperbranched-polyimide-modified epoxy.
resins. Journal of Polymer Science Part B: Polymer Physics. 2006;44(23):3348-3356.
28. Jin F-L, Ma C-J, Park S-J. Thermal and mechanical interfacial properties of epoxy composites based on functionalized carbon nanotubes. Materials Science and Engineering: A. 2011;528(29):8517-8522.
29. Hao Y, Liu F, Han E-H. Protection of epoxy coatings containing polyaniline modified ultra-short glass fibers. Progress in Organic Coatings. 2013;76(4):571-580.
30. Prolongo SG, Meliton BG, Del Rosario G, Ureña A. New alignment procedure of magnetite-CNT hybrid nanofillers on epoxy bulk resin with permanent magnets. Composites Part B: Engineering. 2013;46:166-172.
31. Katariya MN, Jana AK, Parikh PA. Corrosion inhibition effectiveness of zeolite ZSM-5 coating on mild steel against various organic acids and its antimicrobial activity. Journal of Industrial and Engineering Chemistry.

2013;19(1):286-291.
32. INRS. Diglycidyl ether of bisphenol A. Fiche toxicologique n°323. 2020. p. 20.
33. Kim WB, Joshi UA, Lee JS. Making polycarbonates without employing phosgene: An overview on catalytic chemistry of intermediate and precursor syntheses for polycarbonate. Industrial & engineering chemistry research. 2004;43(9):1897-1914.
34. INRS. Plastics, risk and thematic analysis: Polycarbonate PC. 2017. p. 4.
35. Graziani NS, Carreras H, Wannaz E. Atmospheric levels of BPA associated with particulate matter in an urban environment. Heliyon. 2019;5(4):e01419.
36. Liu J, Zhang L, Lu G, Jiang R, Yan Z, Li Y. Occurrence, toxicity and ecological risk of Bisphenol A analogues in aquatic environment - A review. Ecotoxicology and environmental safety. 2021;208:111481.
37. Canada E. Draft screening assessment report for the Challenge related to 4,4'-isopropylidenediphenol (bisphenol A) Chemical Abstracts Service Registry Number 80-05-7La Voie verte. 2008. p. 192.
38. Wang Q, Chen M, Shan G, Chen P, Cui S, Yi S, et al. Bioaccumulation and biomagnification of emerging bisphenol analogues in aquatic organisms from Taihu Lake, China. Science of the Total Environment. 2017;598:814-820.
39. Ji M-K, Kabra AN, Choi J, Hwang J-H, Kim JR, Abou-Shanab RA, et al. Biodegradation of bisphenol A by the freshwater microalgae Chlamydomonas mexicana and Chlorella vulgaris. Ecological engineering. 2014;73:260-269.
40. Zhu Q, Jia J, Wang Y, Zhang K, Zhang H, Liao C, et al. Spatial distribution of parabens, triclocarban, triclosan, bisphenols, and tetrabromobisphenol A and its alternatives in municipal sewage sludges in China. Science of the Total Environment. 2019;679:61-69.
41. Corrales J, Kristofco LA, Steele WB, Yates BS, Breed CS, Williams ES,

et al. Global assessment of bisphenol A in the environment: review and analysis of its occurrence and bioaccumulation. Dose-response. 2015;13(3):1559325815598308.
42. EFSA Panel on Food Contact Materials E, Flavourings, Aids P. Scientific Opinion on the risks to public health related to the presence of bisphenol A (BPA) in foodstuffs. EFSA Journal. 2015;13(1):3978.
43. EFSA Panel on Food Contact Materials E, Aids P, Lambré C, Barat Baviera JM, Bolognesi C, Chesson A, et al. Re-evaluation of the risks to public health related to the presence of bisphenol A (BPA) in foodstuffs. EFSA Journal. 2023;21(4):e06857.
44. Leung Y-K. A Silent Threat: Exploring the Impact of Endocrine Disruption on Human Health. International journal of molecular sciences. 2023;24(12):9790.
45. Commission Regulation (EU) No 10/2011 of 14/01/11 on plastic materials and articles intended to come into contact with foodstuffs, (2011).
46. Canada Consumer Product Safety Act, (2010).
47. EFSA. Opinion of the Scientific Panel on food additives, flavourings, processing aids and materials in contact with food (AFC) related to 2,2-BIS(4-HYDROXYPHENYL)PROPANE. UFSA JOURNAL. 2006:75.
48. Kadasala NR, Narayanan B, Liu Y. International trade regulations on BPA: Global health and economic implications. Asian Development Policy Review. 2016;4(4):134-142.
49. Tarafdar A, Sirohi R, Balakumaran PA, Reshmy R, Madhavan A, Sindhu R, et al. The hazardous threat of Bisphenol A: Toxicity, detection and remediation. Journal of hazardous materials. 2022;423:127097.
50. People's Democratic Republic of Algeria. Arreté interministériel du 6 Chaoual 1437 correspondant au 11 juillet 2016 portant adoption du règlement technique fixant les exigences de sécurité des articles de puériculture., 68 (2016).
51. Corbel T. Toxicokinetic mechanisms involved in fetal exposure to

bisphenol A. Toulouse: Université Toulouse III - Paul Sabatier; 2013.
52. Kawamura Y, Inoue K, Nakazawa H, Yamada T, Maitani T. Cause of bisphenol A migration from cans for drinks and assessment of improved cans. Shokuhin eiseigaku zasshi Journal of the Food Hygienic Society of Japan. 2001;42(1):13-17.
53. Munguia-Lopez EM, Soto-Valdez H. Effect of heat processing and storage time on migration of bisphenol A (BPA) and bisphenol A- diglycidyl ether (BADGE) to aqueous food simulant from Mexican can coatings. Journal of agricultural and food chemistry. 2001;49(8):3666-3671.
54. Cao X-L, Corriveau J, Popovic S. Migration of bisphenol A from can coatings to liquid infant formula during storage at room temperature. Journal of food protection. 2009;72(12):2571-2574.
55. Biles J, McNeal T, Begley T, Hollifield H. Determination of bisphenol-A in reusable polycarbonate food-contact plastics and migration to food-simulating liquids. Journal of agricultural and food chemistry. 1997;45(9):3541-3544.
56. Benhamada M, Bouzid D, Boyron O, Taam M. The relationship between the aging of polycarbonate characterized by SEC and the release of bisphenol A quantified by HPLC-UV. European Food Research and Technology. 2016;242:227-232.
57. Biedermann-Brem S, Grob K, Fjeldal P. Release of bisphenol A from polycarbonate baby bottles: mechanisms of formation and investigation of worst case scenarios. European Food Research and Technology. 2008;227:1053-1060.
58. Yonekubo J, Hayakawa K, Sajiki J. Concentrations of bisphenol A, bisphenol A diglycidyl ether, and their derivatives in canned foods in Japanese markets. Journal of agricultural and food chemistry. 2008;56(6):2041-2047.
59. Munguia-Lopez EM, Peralta E, Gonzalez-Leon A, Vargas-Requena C, Soto-Valdez H. Migration of bisphenol A (BPA) from epoxy can coatings to

jalapeno peppers and an acid food simulant. Journal of agricultural and food chemistry. 2002;50(25):7299-7302.
60. Santillana M, Ruiz E, Nieto M, Rodríguez Bernaldo de Quirós A, Sendón R, Cirugeda M, et al. Polycarbonate baby bottles: study of the release of Bisphenol A. European Food Research and Technology. 2013;236:883-889.
61. Johnson S, Saxena P, Sahu R. Leaching of bisphenol A from baby bottles. Proceedings of the National Academy of Sciences, India Section B: Biological Sciences. 2015;85:131-135.
62. Khalili Sadrabad E, Hashemi SA, Nadjarzadeh A, Askari E, Akrami Mohajeri F, Ramroudi F. Bisphenol A release from food and beverage containers-A review. Food science & nutrition. 2023;11(7):3718 - 3728.
63. Gunatilake SR, Munasinghe VK, Ranaweera R, Mlsna TE, Xia K. Recent advancements in analytical methods for the determination of steroidal estrogen residues in environmental and food matrices. Analytical Methods. 2016;8(28):5556-5568.
64. Varelis P, Balafas D. Preparation of 4, 4'-(1-[2H6] methylethylidene) bis-[2, 3, 5, 6-2H4] phenol and its application to the measurement of bisphenol A in beverages by stable isotope dilution mass spectrometry. Journal of Chromatography A. 2000;883(1-2):163-170.
65. Goodson A, Summerfield W, Cooper I. Survey of bisphenol A and bisphenol F in canned foods. Food Additives & Contaminants. 2002;19(8):796-802.
66. Ballesteros-Gómez A, Rubio S, Pérez-Bendito D. Analytical methods for the determination of bisphenol A in food. Journal of Chromatography A. 2009;1216(3):449-69.
67. Cao X-L. A review recent development on analytical methods for determination of bisphenol a in food and biological samples. Journal of liquid chromatography & related technologies. 2012;35(19):2795-2829.
68. Sun C, Leong LP, Barlow PJ, Chan SH, Bloodworth BC. Single

laboratory validation of a method for the determination of Bisphenol A, Bisphenol A diglycidyl ether and its derivatives in canned foods by reversed-phase liquid chromatography. Journal of Chromatography A. 2006;1129(1):145-148.
69. Liu Y, Wang S, Wang L. Development of rapid determination of 18 phthalate esters in edible vegetable oils by gas chromatography tandem mass spectrometry. Journal of agricultural and food chemistry. 2013;61(6):1160-1164.
70. Lopez-Cervantes J, Paseiro-Losada P. Determination of bisphenol A in, and its migration from, PVC stretch film used for food packaging. Food Additives & Contaminants. 2003;20(6):596-606.
71. Munguia-Lopez E, Gerardo-Lugo S, Peralta E, Bolumen S, Soto-Valdez H. Migration of bisphenol A (BPA) from can coatings into a fatty-food simulant and tuna fish. Food additives and contaminants. 2005;22(9):892-898.
72. Casajuana N, Lacorte S. New methodology for the determination of phthalate esters, bisphenol A, bisphenol A diglycidyl ether, and nonylphenol in commercial whole milk samples. Journal of agricultural and food chemistry. 2004;52(12):3702-3707.
73. Kuo H-W, Ding W-H. Trace determination of bisphenol A and phytoestrogens in infant formula powders by gas chromatography-mass spectrometry. Journal of Chromatography A. 2004;1027(1-2):67-74.
74. Xu D-P, Zou Z-F, Li S, Li H-B, Chen Y-H, Xu X-R. Toxicity, Occurrence and Analytical Method of Bisphenol
A. International Journal of Food Nutrition and . 2013;4(1):1-16.
75. Braunrath R, Podlipna D, Padlesak S, Cichna-Markl M. Determination of bisphenol A in canned foods by immunoaffinity chromatography, HPLC, and fluorescence detection. Journal of agricultural and food chemistry. 2005;53(23):8911-8917.
76. Li Y, Zhang S, Song C, You J. Determination of bisphenol A and

alkylphenols in soft drinks by high-performance liquid chromatography with fluorescence detection. Food Analytical Methods. 2013;6:1284-1290.
77. Vilarinho F, Lestido-Cardama A, Sendón R, Rodríguez Bernaldo de Quirós A, Vaz MdF, Sanches-Silva A. HPLC with fluorescence detection for determination of bisphenol A in canned vegetables: Optimization, validation and application to samples from Portuguese and Spanish markets. Coatings. 2020;10(7):624.
78. Xing J, Zhang S, Zhang M, Hou J. A critical review of presence, removal and potential impacts of endocrine disruptors bisphenol A. Comparative Biochemistry and Physiology Part C: Toxicology & Pharmacology. 2022;254:109275.
79. Lei K, Pan H-Y, Zhu Y, Chen W, Lin C-Y. Pollution characteristics and mixture risk prediction of phenolic environmental estrogens in rivers of the Beijing-Tianjin-Hebei urban agglomeration, China. Science of the Total Environment. 2021;787:147646.
80. Xue J, Kannan K. Mass flows and removal of eight bisphenol analogs, bisphenol A diglycidyl ether and its derivatives in two wastewater treatment plants in New York State, USA. Science of the Total Environment. 2019;648:442- 449.
81. Stachel B, Ehrhorn U, Heemken O-P, Lepom P, Reincke H, Sawal G, et al. Xenoestrogens in the River Elbe and its tributaries. Environmental Pollution. 2003;124(3):497-507.
82. Yamazaki E, Yamashita N, Taniyasu S, Lam J, Lam PK, Moon H-B, et al. Bisphenol A and other bisphenol analogues including BPS and BPF in surface water samples from Japan, China, Korea and India. Ecotoxicology and environmental safety. 2015;122:565-572.
83. Farounbi AI, Ngqwala NP. Occurrence of selected endocrine disrupting compounds in the eastern cape province of South Africa. Environmental Science and Pollution Research. 2020;27(14):17268-17279.
84. Shehab ZN, Jamil NR, Aris AZ. Occurrence, environmental implications

and risk assessment of Bisphenol A in association with colloidal particles in an urban tropical river in Malaysia. Scientific reports. 2020;10(1):20360.

85. Safakhah N, Ghanemi K, Nikpour Y, Batvandi Z. Occurrence, distribution, and risk assessment of bisphenol A in the surface sediments of Musa estuary and its tributaries in the northern end of the Persian Gulf, Iran. Marine pollution bulletin. 2020;156:111241.

86. Fu P, Kawamura K. Ubiquity of bisphenol A in the atmosphere. Environmental Pollution. 2010;158(10):3138- 3143.

87. Salgueiro-González N, Lopez de Alda M, Muniategui-Lorenzo S, Prada-Rodríguez D, Barceló D. Determination of 13 estrogenic endocrine disrupting compounds in atmospheric particulate matter by pressurised liquid extraction and liquid chromatography-tandem mass spectrometry. Analytical and bioanalytical chemistry. 2013;405:8913-8923.

88. Duong HT, Kadokami K, Trinh HT, Phan TQ, Le GT, Nguyen DT, et al. Target screening analysis of 970 semi-volatile organic compounds adsorbed on atmospheric particulate matter in Hanoi, Vietnam. Chemosphere. 2019;219:784- 795.

89. Ferrey ML, Hamilton MC, Backe WJ, Anderson KE. Pharmaceuticals and other anthropogenic chemicals in atmospheric particulates and precipitation. Science of the Total Environment. 2018;612:1488-1497.

90. Kouidhi W, Thannimalay L, Soon CS, Ali Mohd M. Occupational exposure to bisphenol A (BPA) in a plastic injection molding factory in Malaysia. International journal of occupational medicine and environmental health. 2017;30(5):743-750.

91. Hines CJ, Jackson MV, Christianson AL, Clark JC, Arnold JE, Pretty JR, et al. Air, hand wipe, and surface wipe sampling for Bisphenol A (BPA) among workers in industries that manufacture and use BPA in the United States. Journal of Occupational and Environmental Hygiene. 2017;14(11):882-897.

92. Vasiljevic T, Harner T. Bisphenol A and its analogues in outdoor and

indoor air: Properties, sources and global levels. Science of the Total Environment. 2021;789:148013.
93. Liao C, Kannan K. A survey of alkylphenols, bisphenols, and triclosan in personal care products from China and the United States. Archives of environmental contamination and toxicology. 2014;67:50-59.
94. Lu S, Yu Y, Ren L, Zhang X, Liu G, Yu Y. Estimation of intake and uptake of bisphenols and triclosan from personal care products by dermal contact. Science of the Total Environment. 2018;621:1389-1396.
95. Gao C-J, Kannan K. Phthalates, bisphenols, parabens, and triclocarban in feminine hygiene products from the United States and their implications for human exposure. Environment international. 2020;136:105465.
96. Heinälä M, Ylinen K, Tuomi T, Santonen T, Porras SP. Assessment of occupational exposure to bisphenol A in five different production companies in Finland. Annals of work exposures and health. 2017;61(1):44-55.
97. Björnsdotter MK, de Boer J, Ballesteros-Gómez A. Bisphenol A and replacements in thermal paper: A review. Chemosphere. 2017;182:691-706.
98. Wang X, Nag R, Brunton NP, Siddique MAB, Harrison SM, Monahan FJ, et al. Human health risk assessment of bisphenol A (BPA) through meat products. Environmental research. 2022;213:113734.
99. Bemrah N, Jean J, Rivière G, Sanaa M, Leconte S, Bachelot M, et al. Assessment of dietary exposure to bisphenol A in the French population with a special focus on risk characterisation for pregnant French women. Food and Chemical Toxicology. 2014;72:90-7.
100. Gorecki S, Bemrah N, Roudot A-C, Marchioni E, Le Bizec B, Faivre F, et al. Human health risks related to the consumption of foodstuffs of animal origin contaminated by bisphenol A. Food and Chemical Toxicology. 2017;110:333- 339.
101. González N, Cunha SC, Ferreira R, Fernandes JO, Marquès M, Nadal M, et al. Concentrations of nine bisphenol analogues in food purchased from Catalonia (Spain): Comparison of canned and non-canned foodstuffs. Food

and Chemical Toxicology. 2020;136:110992.
102. Ni L, Zhong J, Chi H, Lin N, Liu Z. Recent Advances in Sources, Migration, Public Health, and Surveillance of Bisphenol A and Its Structural Analogs in Canned Foods. Foods. 2023;12(10):1989.
103. Thomson B, Grounds P. Bisphenol A in canned foods in New Zealand: an exposure assessment. Food additives and contaminants. 2005;22(1):65-72.
104. Cao X-L, Corriveau J, Popovic S. Bisphenol A in canned food products from Canadian markets. Journal of food protection. 2010;73(6):1085-1089.
105. van Leeuwen SP, Bovee TF, Awchi M, Klijnstra MD, Hamers AR, Hoogenboom RL, et al. BPA, BADGE and analogues: A new multi-analyte LC-ESI-MS/MS method for their determination and their in vitro (anti) estrogenic and (anti) androgenic properties. Chemosphere. 2019;221:246-253.
106. Adeyi AA, Babalola BA. Bisphenol-A (BPA) in Foods commonly consumed in Southwest Nigeria and its Human Health Risk. Scientific reports. 2019;9(1):17458.
107. Cao P, Zhong H-n, Qiu K, Li D, Wu G, Sui H-x, et al. Exposure to bisphenol A and its substitutes, bisphenol F and bisphenol S from canned foods and beverages on Chinese market. Food Control. 2021;120:107502.
108. Geens T, Aerts D, Berthot C, Bourguignon J-P, Goeyens L, Lecomte P, et al. A review of dietary and non-dietary exposure to bisphenol-A. Food and Chemical Toxicology. 2012;50(10):3725-3740.
109. Hines CJ, Jackson MV, Deddens JA, Clark JC, Ye X, Christianson AL, et al. Urinary bisphenol A (BPA) concentrations among workers in industries that manufacture and use BPA in the USA. Annals of work exposures and health. 2017;61(2):164-182.
110. Thayer KA, Doerge DR, Hunt D, Schurman SH, Twaddle NC, Churchwell MI, et al. Pharmacokinetics of bisphenol A in humans following a single oral administration. Environment international. 2015;83:107-115.

111. Teeguarden JG, Twaddle NC, Churchwell MI, Yang X, Fisher JW, Seryak LM, et al. 24-hour human urine and serum profiles of bisphenol A: Evidence against sublingual absorption following ingestion in soup. Toxicology and applied pharmacology. 2015;288(2):131-142.
112. Sasso AF, Pirow R, Andra SS, Church R, Nachman RM, Linke S, et al. Pharmacokinetics of bisphenol A in humans following dermal administration. Environment international. 2020;144:106031.
113. Collet SH, Picard-Hagen N, Lacroix MZ, Puel S, Viguié C, Bousquet-Melou A, et al. Allometric scaling for predicting human clearance of bisphenol A. Toxicology and applied pharmacology. 2015;284(3):323-329.
114. Csanády G, Oberste-Frielinghaus H, Semder B, Baur C, Schneider K, Filser J. Distribution and unspecific protein binding of the xenoestrogens bisphenol A and daidzein. Archives of toxicology. 2002;76:299-305.
115. Déchaud H, Ravard C, Claustrat F, de la Perrière AB, Pugeat M. Xenoestrogen interaction with human sex hormone-binding globulin (hSHBG) 1. Steroids. 1999;64(5):328-334.
116. Gramec Skledar D, Peterlin Masic L. Bisphenol A and its analogs: Do their metabolites have endocrine activity?
Environmental toxicology and pharmacology. 2016;47:182-199.
117. Ramírez V, Gálvez-Ontiveros Y, Porras-Quesada P, Martinez-Gonzalez LJ, Rivas A, Álvarez-Cubero MJ. Metabolic pathways, alterations in miRNAs expression and effects of genetic polymorphisms of bisphenol a analogues: A systematic review. Environmental research. 2021;197:111062.
118. Provencher G, Bérubé R, Dumas P, Bienvenu J-F, Gaudreau É, Bélanger P, et al. Determination of bisphenol A, triclosan and their metabolites in human urine using isotope-dilution liquid chromatography-tandem mass spectrometry. Journal of Chromatography A. 2014;1348:97-104.
119. Okuda K, Takiguchi M, Yoshihara Si. In vivo estrogenic potential of 4-methyl-2, 4-bis (4-hydroxyphenyl) pent- 1-ene, an active metabolite of

bisphenol A, in uterus of ovariectomized rat. Toxicology letters. 2010;197(1):7-11.
120. Nakamura S, Tezuka Y, Ushiyama A, Kawashima C, Kitagawara Y, Takahashi K, et al. Ipso substitution of bisphenol A catalyzed by microsomal cytochrome P450 and enhancement of estrogenic activity. Toxicology letters. 2011;203(1):92-95.
121. Wisniowska B, Linke S, Polak S, Bielecka Z, Luch A, Pirow R. Data on ADME parameters of bisphenol A and
its metabolites for use in physiologically based pharmacokinetic modelling. Data in brief. 2023;48:109101.
122. Cimmino I, Fiory F, Perruolo G, Miele C, Beguinot F, Formisano P, et al. Potential mechanisms of bisphenol A (BPA) contributing to human disease. International journal of molecular sciences. 2020;21(16):5761.
123. Tyl R, Myers C, Marr M, Thomas B, Keimowitz A, Brine D, et al. Three-generation reproductive toxicity study of dietary bisphenol A in CD Sprague-Dawley rats. Toxicological Sciences. 2002;68(1):121-146.
124. Oguazu CE, Ezeonu FC, Ubaoji KI, Anajekwu B. Bisphol a exerts a transient perturbation of liver function in wistar albino rats at acute and sub-chronic exposure doses. Journal of Pharmacological Science and Bioscientific Research. 2015;5(3):274-278.
125. Tyl RW, Myers CB, Marr MC, Sloan CS, Castillo NP, Veselica MM, et al. Two-generation reproductive toxicity study of dietary bisphenol A in CD-1 (Swiss) mice. Toxicological Sciences. 2008;104(2):362-384.
126. Ke Z-H, Pan J-X, Jin L-Y, Xu H-Y, Yu T-T, Ullah K, et al. Bisphenol A exposure may induce hepatic lipid accumulation via reprogramming the DNA methylation patterns of genes involved in lipid metabolism. Scientific reports. 2016;6(1):31331.
127. Rezg R, El-Fazaa S, Gharbi N, Mornagui B. Bisphenol A and human chronic diseases: current evidences, possible mechanisms, and future perspectives. Environment international. 2014;64:83-90.

128. Li D-K, Zhou Z, Miao M, He Y, Wang J, Ferber J, et al. Urine bisphenol-A (BPA) level in relation to semen quality. Fertility and Sterility. 2011;95(2):625-30.e4.
129. Zhou Q, Miao M, Ran M, Ding L, Bai L, Wu T, et al. Serum bisphenol-A concentration and sex hormone levels in men. Fertility and Sterility. 2013;100(2):478-482.
130. Ehrlich S, Williams PL, Missmer SA, Flaws JA, Berry KF, Calafat AM, et al. Urinary bisphenol A concentrations and implantation failure among women undergoing in vitro fertilization. Environmental health perspectives. 2012;120(7):978-983.
131. Bloom MS, Vom Saal FS, Kim D, Taylor JA, Lamb JD, Fujimoto VY. Serum unconjugated bisphenol A concentrations in men may influence embryo quality indicators during in vitro fertilization. Environmental toxicology and pharmacology. 2011;32(2):319-323.
132. Tarantino G, Valentino R, Somma CD, D'Esposito V, Passaretti F, Pizza G, et al. Bisphenol A in polycystic ovary syndrome and its association with liver-spleen axis. Clinical endocrinology. 2013;78(3):447-453.
133. Itoh H, Iwasaki M, Hanaoka T, Sasaki H, Tanaka T, Tsugane S. Urinary bisphenol-A concentration in infertile Japanese women and its association with endometriosis: A cross-sectional study. Environmental health and preventive medicine. 2007;12(6):258-264.
134. Miao M, Yuan W, Zhu G, He X, Li D-K. In utero exposure to bisphenol-A and its effect on birth weight of offspring. Reproductive toxicology. 2011;32(1):64-68.
135. Braun JM, Yolton K, Dietrich KN, Hornung R, Ye X, Calafat AM, et al. Prenatal bisphenol A exposure and early childhood behavior. Environmental health perspectives. 2009;117(12):1945-1952.
136. Perera F, Vishnevetsky J, Herbstman JB, Calafat AM, Xiong W, Rauh V, et al. Prenatal bisphenol a exposure and child behavior in an inner-city cohort. Environmental health perspectives. 2012;120(8):1190-1194.

137. Miao M, Yuan W, He Y, Zhou Z, Wang J, Gao E, et al. In utero exposure to bisphenol-A and anogenital distance of male offspring. Birth Defects Research Part A: Clinical and Molecular Teratology. 2011;91(10):867-872.
138. Fenichel P, Dechaux H, Harthe C, Gal J, Ferrari P, Pacini P, et al. Unconjugated bisphenol A cord blood levels in boys with descended or undescended testes. Human reproduction. 2012;27(4):983-990.
139. Melzer D, Osborne NJ, Henley WE, Cipelli R, Young A, Money C, et al. Urinary bisphenol A concentration and risk of future coronary artery disease in apparently healthy men and women. Circulation. 2012;125(12):1482-1490.
140. Olsen L, Lind L, Lind PM. Associations between circulating levels of bisphenol A and phthalate metabolites and coronary risk in the elderly. Ecotoxicology and environmental safety. 2012;80:179-183.
141. Lang IA, Galloway TS, Scarlett A, Henley WE, Depledge M, Wallace RB, et al. Association of urinary bisphenol A concentration with medical disorders and laboratory abnormalities in adults. Jama. 2008;300(11):1303-1310.
142. Silver MK, O'Neill MS, Sowers MR, Park SK. Urinary bisphenol A and type-2 diabetes in US adults: data from NHANES 2003-2008. PloS one. 2011;6(10):e26868.
143. Wang F, Hua J, Chen M, Xia Y, Zhang Q, Zhao R, et al. High urinary bisphenol A concentrations in workers and possible laboratory abnormalities. Occupational and environmental medicine. 2012;69(9):679-684.
144. Chevrier J, Gunier RB, Bradman A, Holland NT, Calafat AM, Eskenazi B, et al. Maternal urinary bisphenol a during pregnancy and maternal and neonatal thyroid function in the CHAMACOS study. Environmental health perspectives. 2013;121(1):138-144.
145. Brucker-Davis F, Ferrari P, Boda-Buccino M, Wagner-Mahler K,

Pacini P, Gal J, et al. Cord blood thyroid tests in boys born with and without cryptorchidism: correlations with birth parameters and in utero xenobiotics exposure. Thyroid. 2011;21(10):1133-1141.
146. Xu J, Huang G, Guo TL. Developmental Bisphenol A Exposure Modulates Immune-Related Diseases. Toxics. 2016;4(4):23.
147. Hess-Wilson JK, Webb SL, Daly HK, Leung Y-K, Boldison J, Comstock CE, et al. Unique bisphenol A transcriptome in prostate cancer: Novel effects on ERB expression that correspond to androgen receptor mutation status. Environmental health perspectives. 2007;115(11):1646-1653.
148. Morgan M, Deoraj A, Felty Q, Yoo C, Roy D. Association between exposure to estrogenic endocrine disruptors- polychlorinated biphenyls, phthalates, and bisphenol A and gynecologic cancers-cervical, ovarian, uterine cancers. Journal of Carcinogenesis & Mutagenesis. 2016;7(6):1000275.
149. Prueitt RL, Hixon ML, Fan T, Olgun NS, Piatos P, Zhou J, et al. Systematic review of the potential carcinogenicity of bisphenol A in humans. Regulatory Toxicology and Pharmacology. 2023;142:105414.
150. Manzoor MF, Tariq T, Fatima B, Sahar A, Tariq F, Munir S, et al. An insight into bisphenol A, food exposure and its adverse effects on health: A review. Frontiers in nutrition. 2022;9:1047827.
151. Chen D, Kannan K, Tan H, Zheng Z, Feng Y-L, Wu Y, et al. Bisphenol analogues other than BPA: environmental occurrence, human exposure, and toxicity: a review. Environmental science & technology. 2016;50(11):5438-5453.
152. Pelch K, Wignall JA, Goldstone AE, Ross PK, Blain RB, Shapiro AJ, et al. A scoping review of the health and toxicological activity of bisphenol A (BPA) structural analogues and functional alternatives. Toxicology. 2019;424:152235.
153. Liao C, Liu F, Moon H-B, Yamashita N, Yun S, Kannan K. Bisphenol

analogues in sediments from industrialized areas in the United States, Japan, and Korea: spatial and temporal distributions. Environmental science & technology. 2012;46(21):11558-11565.

154. Song S, Song M, Zeng L, Wang T, Liu R, Ruan T, et al. Occurrence and profiles of bisphenol analogues in municipal sewage sludge in China. Environmental Pollution. 2014;186:14-19.

155. Grumetto L, Montesano D, Seccia S, Albrizio S, Barbato F. Determination of bisphenol A and bisphenol B residues in canned peeled tomatoes by reversed-phase liquid chromatography. Journal of agricultural and food chemistry. 2008;56(22):10633-10637.

156. Liao C, Kannan K. Concentrations and profiles of bisphenol A and other bisphenol analogues in foodstuffs from the United States and their implications for human exposure. Journal of agricultural and food chemistry. 2013;61(19):4655-4662.

157. Viñas P, Campillo N, Martínez-Castillo N, Hernández-Córdoba M. Comparison of two derivatization-based methods for solid-phase microextraction-gas chromatography-mass spectrometric determination of bisphenol A, bisphenol S and biphenol migrated from food cans. Analytical and bioanalytical chemistry. 2010;397:115-125.

158. Asimakopoulos AG, Xue J, De Carvalho BP, Iyer A, Abualnaja KO, Yaghmoor SS, et al. Urinary biomarkers of exposure to 57 xenobiotics and its association with oxidative stress in a population in Jeddah, Saudi Arabia. Environmental research. 2016;150:573-581.

159. Yang Y, Shi Y, Chen D, Chen H, Liu X. Bisphenol A and its analogues in paired urine and house dust from South China and implications for children's exposure. Chemosphere. 2022;294:133701.

160. Jurewicz J, Majewska J, Berg A, Owczarek K, Zajdel R, Kaleta D, et al. Serum bisphenol A analogues in women diagnosed with the polycystic ovary syndrome-is there an association? Environmental Pollution. 2021;272:115962.

161. Rochester JR, Bolden AL. Bisphenol S and F: a systematic review and comparison of the hormonal activity of bisphenol A substitutes. Environmental health perspectives. 2015;123(7):643-650.
162. Sendra M, Stampar M, Fras K, Novoa B, Figueras A, Zegura B. Adverse (geno) toxic effects of bisphenol A and its analogues in hepatic 3D cell model. Environment international. 2023;171:107721.

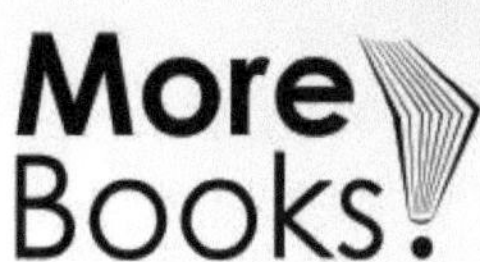

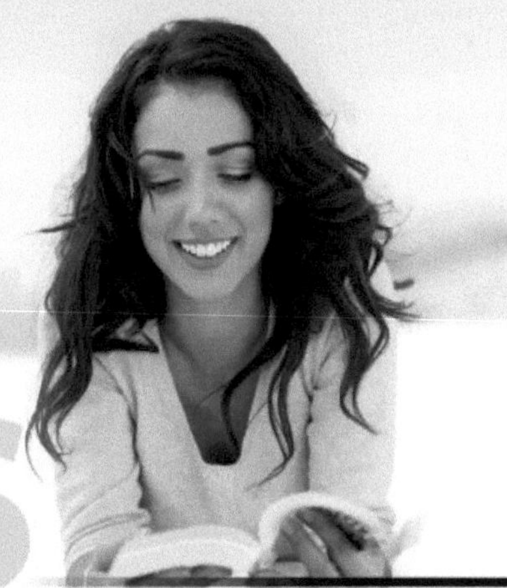

yes

I want morebooks!

Buy your books fast and straightforward online - at one of world's fastest growing online book stores! Environmentally sound due to Print-on-Demand technologies.

Buy your books online at
www.morebooks.shop

Kaufen Sie Ihre Bücher schnell und unkompliziert online – auf einer der am schnellsten wachsenden Buchhandelsplattformen weltweit! Dank Print-On-Demand umwelt- und ressourcenschonend produzi ert.

Bücher schneller online kaufen
www.morebooks.shop

info@omniscriptum.com
www.omniscriptum.com

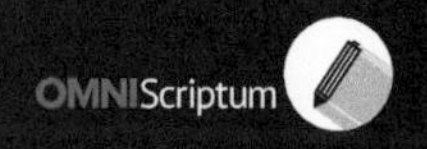

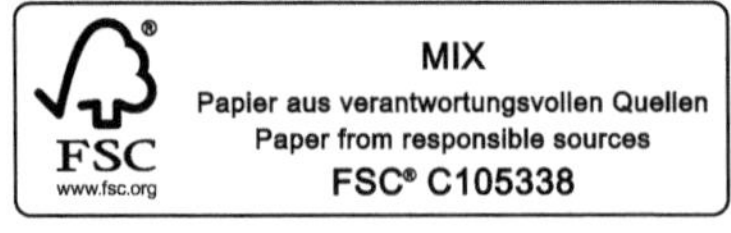

Printed by Books on Demand GmbH, Norderstedt / Germany